My Nutrition Log

Making Better Choices

Right Track Publishing

Olathe, KS

My Nutrition Log: Making Better Choices
The Fervent Fermenter Series
Published by Right Track Publishing in 2017
righttrackpublishing.com

The information provided in this publication is for educational and record-keeping purposes only, and is not intended to replace professional medical or nutritional advice. For best results, make small, incremental, realistic changes. And always consult your doctor when making dietary or lifestyle changes that could affect your health.

ISBN: 978-0-9913371-8-7

Making Better Choices

Do you feel lethargic, bloated, and just plain yucky most of the time? Did you ever go without sugar or junk food for a week and start to feel better? Most Americans know their diets are awful. We lead busy lives. It seems easier to grab fast food or rely on processed foods for quicker meals than it is to plan, prepare, and take a little extra time for cooking. Yet, we feel blah and drag through each day with little mental and physical energy.

We know we need to make changes, but it sometimes feels overwhelming and complicated. The good news is that it doesn't have to be! You might not be able to do *everything* at once, but you can do *something* at once; just one or two changes at a time. Let your new mantra be: "Out with the bad, in with the good."

Make the switch! Switch sugar for stevia, sparkling water for soda, cereal for steel-cut oats, transfats for medium-chain healthy fats, and try to buy cuts of meat from grass-fed cows and free-range chickens when possible. When you remove an unhealthy food from your diet, don't leave a void; replace it with something better.

Be a learner! Read up on the benefits of juicing, green smoothies, raw and fermented foods, and organic eating. Get active. Add some movement if you live a sedentary lifestyle. Periodic stretching throughout the day, taking the stairs instead of the elevator, and walking more are steps in the right direction!

Finally, make sure you drink enough good quality water. Think about investing in a reverse osmosis water system or filling up a couple 5-gallon jugs each week at Whole Foods Market or someplace with a water filtering station. As they say, "Use a filter or be a filter."

The resources below have good information and recipes!

Books

Grain Brain: The Surprising Truth about Wheat, Carbs, and Sugar--Your Brain's Silent Killers
by David Perlmutter (with Kristen Loberg)

That Sugar Book: This Book Will Change the Way You Think About 'Healthy' Food
by Damon Gameau

Raw and Simple: Eat Well and Live Radiantly with 100 Truly Quick and Easy Recipes for the Raw Food Lifestyle
by Judith Wignall

Eat Happy: Gluten Free, Grain Free, Low Carb Recipes Made from Real Foods For A Joyful Life
by Anna Vocino

The Juice Lover's Big Book of Juices: 425 Recipes for Super Nutritious and Crazy Delicious Juices
by Vanessa Simkins

How to Use This Journal

Keep this on your kitchen counter or nightstand and track your progress daily!

Calendars: Jot the days of the month in the appropriate squares. Choose two colored pencils or crayons. On the days you achieve your goals, color the square in with your favorite color. On days you don't meet your goals, fill in the square with the other color. You will be able to see at a glance how many days of success you're having each month. Hopefully, each month will be better than the last!

Daily Tracking: What things do you want to cut back on? Sugar? Salt? Gluten? Caffeine? Alcohol? Simple carbs? Meat? Dairy?

What things do you want to add? Fermented foods? Raw foods? Juicing? Smoothies? Vitamins or other supplements? Drinking more water? Green tea?

What are you eating for breakfast, lunch, and dinner; or are you skipping meals? Are you having regular bowel movements? At the end of the day how do you feel? Keeping track of what you eat and drink throughout the day, and then observing how you feel at bedtime, will help you know your body better.

Notes: Write down any physical symptoms you have, both the good and bad, like: headaches, cramps, indigestion, and fatigue; or more energy, clearer mind, improved complexion, and less pain.

Knowledge acted upon is power. Get to know your body so you can make better nutritional choices that will help you go from feeling gross to feeling great!

Taking Assessment

I struggle with:

- ☐ Weight
- ☐ Brain Fog:
- ☐ Pain
- ☐ Diabetes
- ☐ Low Energy
- ☐ Sleep problems
- ☐ Digestive issues
- ☐ Autoimmune disorder

My biggest health concerns are: ____________

____

____

____

____

____

My reasons for keeping a food diary are::

____

____

____

____

____

My weight goal is: ____________________________

♡ I'm a "Lone Ranger"

♡ I have an accountability partner

Out With the Bad
In With the Good!

I want to eliminate these things from my diet:

I want to add these things to my diet:

I want to include these supplements:

Color _________ = Success!   Color _________ = Not quite

Month _______________

Month _______________

Month ______________

Month ______________

Month ________________

Month ________________

Month ______________

Month ______________

Month ____________

Month ____________

Month ______________

Month ______________

Date: ________ ________ Weight

Daily Details

Today I ate these healthy things:

Today I successfully avoided eating:

I took these supplements:

I Drank this many glasses (8 oz.) of water:

1 2 3 4 5 6 7 8 Other ________

☐ B.M. ☐ No B.M.

☐ Felt blah ☐ Felt good ♡ Felt great!

Breakfast: Calories _______

Lunch: Calories _______

Dinner: Calories _______

Snacks

Beverages

Notes:

Date: ________ ________ Weight

Daily Details

Today I ate these healthy things:

Today I successfully avoided eating:

I took these supplements:

I Drank this many glasses (8 oz.) of water:

1 2 3 4 5 6 7 8 Other ________

☐ B.M. ☐ No B.M.

☐ Felt blah ☐ Felt good ♡ Felt great!

Breakfast: Calories ______

Lunch: Calories ______

Dinner: Calories ______

Snacks

Beverages

Notes:

Date: ________ ________ Weight

Daily Details

Today I ate these healthy things:

Today I successfully avoided eating:

I took these supplements:

I Drank this many glasses (8 oz.) of water:

1 2 3 4 5 6 7 8 Other ______

☐ B.M. ☐ No B.M.

☐ Felt blah ☐ Felt good ♡ Felt great!

Breakfast: Calories ________

Lunch: Calories ________

Dinner: Calories ________

Snacks

Beverages

Notes:

Date: ________ ________ Weight

Daily Details

Today I ate these healthy things:

Today I successfully avoided eating:

I took these supplements:

I Drank this many glasses (8 oz.) of water:

1 2 3 4 5 6 7 8 Other ______

☐ B.M. ☐ No B.M.

☐ Felt blah ☐ Felt good ♡ Felt great!

Breakfast: Calories ______

Lunch: Calories ______

Dinner: Calories ______

Snacks

Beverages

Notes:

Date: ________ ________ Weight

Daily Details

Today I ate these healthy things:

Today I successfully avoided eating:

I took these supplements:

I Drank this many glasses (8 oz.) of water:

1 2 3 4 5 6 7 8 Other ________

☐ B.M. ☐ No B.M.

☐ Felt blah ☐ Felt good ♡ Felt great!

Breakfast: Calories ______

Lunch: Calories ______

Dinner: Calories ______

Snacks

Beverages

Notes:

Date: ________ ________ Weight

Daily Details

Today I ate these healthy things:

Today I successfully avoided eating:

I took these supplements:

I Drank this many glasses (8 oz.) of water:

1 2 3 4 5 6 7 8 Other ______

☐ B.M. ☐ No B.M.

☐ Felt blah ☐ Felt good ♡ Felt great!

Breakfast: Calories ________

Lunch: Calories ________

Dinner: Calories ________

Snacks Beverages

Notes:

Date: ________ ________ Weight

Daily Details

Today I ate these healthy things:

Today I successfully avoided eating:

I took these supplements:

I Drank this many glasses (8 oz.) of water:

1 2 3 4 5 6 7 8 Other ________

☐ B.M. ☐ No B.M.

☐ Felt blah ☐ Felt good ♡ Felt great!

Breakfast: Calories ______

Lunch: Calories ______

Dinner: Calories ______

Snacks

Beverages

Notes:

Date: ________ ________ Weight

Daily Details

Today I ate these healthy things:

Today I successfully avoided eating:

I took these supplements:

I Drank this many glasses (8 oz.) of water:

1 2 3 4 5 6 7 8 Other ________

☐ B.M. ☐ No B.M.

☐ Felt blah ☐ Felt good ♡ Felt great!

Breakfast: Calories _______

Lunch: Calories _______

Dinner: Calories _______

Snacks

Beverages

Notes:

Date: ________ ________ Weight

Daily Details

Today I ate these healthy things:

Today I successfully avoided eating:

I took these supplements:

I Drank this many glasses (8 oz.) of water:

1 2 3 4 5 6 7 8 Other ________

☐ B.M. ☐ No B.M.

☐ Felt blah ☐ Felt good ♡ Felt great!

Breakfast: Calories ________

Lunch: Calories ________

Dinner: Calories ________

Snacks

Beverages

Notes:

Date: ________ ________ Weight

Daily Details

Today I ate these healthy things:

Today I successfully avoided eating:

I took these supplements:

I Drank this many glasses (8 oz.) of water:

1 2 3 4 5 6 7 8 Other ________

☐ B.M. ☐ No B.M.

☐ Felt blah ☐ Felt good ♡ Felt great!

Breakfast: Calories ________

Lunch: Calories ________

Dinner: Calories ________

Snacks

Beverages

Notes:

Date: ________ ________ Weight

Daily Details

Today I ate these healthy things:

Today I successfully avoided eating:

I took these supplements:

I Drank this many glasses (8 oz.) of water:

1 2 3 4 5 6 7 8 Other ________

☐ B.M. ☐ No B.M.

☐ Felt blah ☐ Felt good ♡ Felt great!

Breakfast: Calories ______

Lunch: Calories ______

Dinner: Calories ______

Snacks

Beverages

Notes:

Date: ________ ________ Weight

Daily Details

Today I ate these healthy things:

Today I successfully avoided eating:

I took these supplements:

I Drank this many glasses (8 oz.) of water:

1 2 3 4 5 6 7 8 Other ________

☐ B.M. ☐ No B.M.

☐ Felt blah ☐ Felt good ♡ Felt great!

Breakfast: Calories ______

Lunch: Calories ______

Dinner: Calories ______

Snacks

Beverages

Notes:

Date: ________ ________ Weight

Daily Details

Today I ate these healthy things:

Today I successfully avoided eating:

I took these supplements:

I Drank this many glasses (8 oz.) of water:

1 2 3 4 5 6 7 8 Other ________

☐ B.M. ☐ No B.M.

☐ Felt blah ☐ Felt good ♡ Felt great!

Breakfast: Calories ________

Lunch: Calories ________

Dinner: Calories ________

Snacks

Beverages

Notes:

Date: ________ ________ Weight

Daily Details

Today I ate these healthy things:

Today I successfully avoided eating:

I took these supplements:

I Drank this many glasses (8 oz.) of water:

1 2 3 4 5 6 7 8 Other ________

☐ B.M. ☐ No B.M.

☐ Felt blah ☐ Felt good ♡ Felt great!

Breakfast: Calories ________

Lunch: Calories ________

Dinner: Calories ________

Snacks

Beverages

Notes:

Date: ________ ________ Weight

Daily Details

Today I ate these healthy things:

Today I successfully avoided eating:

I took these supplements:

I Drank this many glasses (8 oz.) of water:

1 2 3 4 5 6 7 8 Other ________

☐ B.M. ☐ No B.M.

☐ Felt blah ☐ Felt good ♡ Felt great!

Breakfast: Calories ________

Lunch: Calories ________

Dinner: Calories ________

Snacks

Beverages

Notes:

Date: ________ ________ Weight

Daily Details

Today I ate these healthy things:

Today I successfully avoided eating:

I took these supplements:

I Drank this many glasses (8 oz.) of water:

1 2 3 4 5 6 7 8 Other ______

☐ B.M. ☐ No B.M.

☐ Felt blah ☐ Felt good ♡ Felt great!

Breakfast: Calories ________

Lunch: Calories ________

Dinner: Calories ________

Snacks

Beverages

Notes:

Date: ________ ________ Weight

Daily Details

Today I ate these healthy things:

Today I successfully avoided eating:

I took these supplements:

I Drank this many glasses (8 oz.) of water:

1 2 3 4 5 6 7 8 Other ________

☐ B.M. ☐ No B.M.

☐ Felt blah ☐ Felt good ♡ Felt great!

Breakfast: Calories ______

Lunch: Calories ______

Dinner: Calories ______

Snacks

Beverages

Notes:

Date: ________ ________ Weight

Daily Details

Today I ate these healthy things:

Today I successfully avoided eating:

I took these supplements:

I Drank this many glasses (8 oz.) of water:

1 2 3 4 5 6 7 8 Other ________

☐ B.M. ☐ No B.M.

☐ Felt blah ☐ Felt good ♡ Felt great!

Breakfast:

Calories ________

Lunch:

Calories ________

Dinner:

Calories ________

Snacks

Beverages

Notes:

Date: ________ ________ Weight

Daily Details

Today I ate these healthy things:

Today I successfully avoided eating:

I took these supplements:

I Drank this many glasses (8 oz.) of water:

1 2 3 4 5 6 7 8 Other ________

☐ B.M. ☐ No B.M.

☐ Felt blah ☐ Felt good ♡ Felt great!

Breakfast: Calories ________

Lunch: Calories ________

Dinner: Calories ________

Snacks

Beverages

Notes:

Date: ________ ________ Weight

Daily Details

Today I ate these healthy things:

Today I successfully avoided eating:

I took these supplements:

I Drank this many glasses (8 oz.) of water:

1 2 3 4 5 6 7 8 Other ________

☐ B.M. ☐ No B.M.

☐ Felt blah ☐ Felt good ♡ Felt great!

Breakfast: Calories ________

Lunch: Calories ________

Dinner: Calories ________

Snacks

Beverages

Notes:

Date: ________ ________ Weight

Daily Details

Today I ate these healthy things:

Today I successfully avoided eating:

I took these supplements:

I Drank this many glasses (8 oz.) of water:

1 2 3 4 5 6 7 8 Other ________

☐ B.M. ☐ No B.M.

☐ Felt blah ☐ Felt good ♡ Felt great!

Breakfast: Calories ________

Lunch: Calories ________

Dinner: Calories ________

Snacks

Beverages

Notes:

Date: ________ ________ Weight

Daily Details

Today I ate these healthy things:

Today I successfully avoided eating:

I took these supplements:

I Drank this many glasses (8 oz.) of water:

1 2 3 4 5 6 7 8 Other ________

☐ B.M. ☐ No B.M.

☐ Felt blah ☐ Felt good ♡ Felt great!

Breakfast: Calories ________

Lunch: Calories ________

Dinner: Calories ________

Snacks

Beverages

Notes:

Date: ________ ________ Weight

Daily Details

Today I ate these healthy things:

Today I successfully avoided eating:

I took these supplements:

I Drank this many glasses (8 oz.) of water:

1 2 3 4 5 6 7 8 Other ________

☐ B.M. ☐ No B.M.

☐ Felt blah ☐ Felt good ♡ Felt great!

Breakfast: Calories ________

Lunch: Calories ________

Dinner: Calories ________

Snacks

Beverages

Notes:

Date: ________ ________ Weight

Daily Details

Today I ate these healthy things:

Today I successfully avoided eating:

I took these supplements:

I Drank this many glasses (8 oz) of water:

1 2 3 4 5 6 7 8 Other ________

☐ B.M. ☐ No B.M.

☐ Felt blah ☐ Felt good ♡ Felt great!

Breakfast: Calories ________

Lunch: Calories ________

Dinner: Calories ________

Snacks

Beverages

Notes:

Date: ________ ________ Weight

Daily Details

Today, I ate these healthy things:

Today, I successfully avoided eating:

I took these supplements:

I Drank this many glasses (8 oz.) of water:

1 2 3 4 5 6 7 8 Other ______

☐ B.M. ☐ No B.M.

☐ Felt blah ☐ Felt good ♡ Felt great!

Breakfast: Calories ________

Lunch: Calories ________

Dinner: Calories ________

Snacks

Beverages

Notes:

Date: ________ ________ Weight

Daily Details

Today I ate these healthy things:

Today I successfully avoided eating:

I took these supplements:

I Drank this many glasses (8 oz.) of water:

1 2 3 4 5 6 7 8 Other ______

☐ B.M. ☐ No B.M.

☐ Felt blah ☐ Felt good ♡ Felt great!

Breakfast: Calories _______

Lunch: Calories _______

Dinner: Calories _______

Snacks

Beverages

Notes:

Date: ________ ________ Weight

Daily Details

Today I ate these healthy things:

Today I successfully avoided eating:

I took these supplements:

I Drank this many glasses (8 oz.) of water:

1 2 3 4 5 6 7 8 Other ________

☐ B.M. ☐ No B.M.

☐ Felt blah ☐ Felt good ♡ Felt great!

Breakfast: Calories _______

Lunch: Calories _______

Dinner: Calories _______

Snacks

Beverages

Notes:

Date: ________ ________ Weight

Daily Details

Today I ate these healthy things:

Today I successfully avoided eating:

I took these supplements:

I Drank this many glasses (8 oz.) of water:

1 2 3 4 5 6 7 8 Other ________

☐ B.M. ☐ No B.M.

☐ Felt blah ☐ Felt good ♡ Felt great!

Breakfast: Calories ________

Lunch: Calories ________

Dinner: Calories ________

Snacks

Beverages

Notes:

Date: ________ ________ Weight

Daily Details

Today I ate these healthy things:

Today I successfully avoided eating:

I took these supplements:

I Drank this many glasses (8 oz.) of water:

1 2 3 4 5 6 7 8 Other ______

☐ B.M. ☐ No B.M.

☐ Felt blah ☐ Felt good ♡ Felt great!

Breakfast: Calories ________

Lunch: Calories ________

Dinner: Calories ________

Snacks

Beverages

Notes:

Date: ________ ________ Weight

Daily Details

Today I ate these healthy things:

Today I successfully avoided eating:

I took these supplements:

I Drank this many glasses (8 oz.) of water:

1 2 3 4 5 6 7 8 Other ________

☐ B.M. ☐ No B.M.

☐ Felt blah ☐ Felt good ♡ Felt great!

Breakfast: Calories ______

Lunch: Calories ______

Dinner: Calories ______

Snacks

Beverages

Notes:

Date: ________ ________ Weight

Daily Details

Today I ate these healthy things:

Today I successfully avoided eating:

I took these supplements:

I Drank this many glasses (8 oz.) of water:

1 2 3 4 5 6 7 8 Other ________

☐ B.M. ☐ No B.M.

☐ Felt blah ☐ Felt good ♡ Felt great!

Breakfast: Calories ________

Lunch: Calories ________

Dinner: Calories ________

Snacks

Beverages

Notes:

Date: ________ ________ Weight

Daily Details

Today I ate these healthy things:

Today I successfully avoided eating:

I took these supplements:

I Drank this many glasses (8 oz.) of water:

1 2 3 4 5 6 7 8 Other ________

☐ B.M. ☐ No B.M.

☐ Felt blah ☐ Felt good ♡ Felt great!

Breakfast: Calories ______

Lunch: Calories ______

Dinner: Calories ______

Snacks

Beverages

Notes:

Date: ________ ________ Weight

Daily Details

Today I ate these healthy things:

Today I successfully avoided eating:

I took these supplements:

I Drank this many glasses (8 oz) of water:

1 2 3 4 5 6 7 8 Other ________

☐ B.M. ☐ No B.M.

☐ Felt blah ☐ Felt good ♡ Felt great!

Breakfast: Calories ________

Lunch: Calories ________

Dinner: Calories ________

Snacks

Beverages

Notes:

Date: ________   ________ Weight

Daily Details

Today I ate these healthy things:

______________________ ______________________

______________________ ______________________

______________________ ______________________

____

Today I successfully avoided eating:

____

____

____

I took these supplements:

____

____

I Drank this many glasses (8 oz.) of water:

1 2 3 4 5 6 7 8 Other ________

☐ B.M. ☐ No B.M.

☐ Felt blah ☐ Felt good ♡ Felt great!

Breakfast: Calories ________

Lunch: Calories ________

Dinner: Calories ________

Snacks

Beverages

Notes:

Date: ________ ________ Weight

Daily Details

Today I ate these healthy things:

Today I successfully avoided eating:

I took these supplements:

I Drank this many glasses (8 oz.) of water:

1 2 3 4 5 6 7 8 Other ______

☐ B.M. ☐ No B.M.

☐ Felt blah ☐ Felt good ♡ Felt great!

Breakfast: Calories ________

Lunch: Calories ________

Dinner: Calories ________

Snacks

Beverages

Notes:

Date: ________ ________ Weight

Daily Details

Today I ate these healthy things:

Today I successfully avoided eating:

I took these supplements:

I Drank this many glasses (8 oz.) of water:

1 2 3 4 5 6 7 8 Other ________

☐ B.M. ☐ No B.M.

☐ Felt blah ☐ Felt good ♡ Felt great!

Breakfast: Calories ________

Lunch: Calories ________

Dinner: Calories ________

Snacks

Beverages

Notes:

Date: ________ ________ Weight

Daily Details

Today I ate these healthy things:

Today I successfully avoided eating:

I took these supplements:

I Drank this many glasses (8 oz.) of water:

1 2 3 4 5 6 7 8 Other ________

☐ B.M. ☐ No B.M.

☐ Felt blah ☐ Felt good ♡ Felt great!

Breakfast: Calories ______

Lunch: Calories ______

Dinner: Calories ______

Snacks

Beverages

Notes:

Date: ________ ________ Weight

Daily Details

Today I ate these healthy things:

Today I successfully avoided eating:

I took these supplements:

I Drank this many glasses (8 oz.) of water:

1 2 3 4 5 6 7 8 Other ________

☐ B.M. ☐ No B.M.

☐ Felt blah ☐ Felt good ♡ Felt great!

Breakfast: Calories ______

Lunch: Calories ______

Dinner: Calories ______

Snacks

Beverages

Notes:

Date: ________ ________ Weight

Daily Details

Today I ate these healthy things:

Today I successfully avoided eating:

I took these supplements:

I Drank this many glasses (8 oz.) of water:

1 2 3 4 5 6 7 8 Other ________

☐ B.M. ☐ No B.M.

☐ Felt blah ☐ Felt good ♡ Felt great!

Breakfast: Calories ________

Lunch: Calories ________

Dinner: Calories ________

Snacks

Beverages

Notes:

Date: ________ ________ Weight

Daily Details

Today I ate these healthy things:

________ ________
________ ________
________ ________
____

Today I successfully avoided eating:

____
____
____

I took these supplements:

____
____

I Drank this many glasses (8 oz.) of water:

1 2 3 4 5 6 7 8 Other ________

☐ B.M. ☐ No B.M.

☐ Felt blah ☐ Felt good ♡ Felt great!

Breakfast: Calories ________

Lunch: Calories ________

Dinner: Calories ________

Snacks

Beverages

Notes:

Date: ________ ________ Weight

Daily Details

Today I ate these healthy things:

Today I successfully avoided eating:

I took these supplements:

I Drank this many glasses (8 oz.) of water:

1 2 3 4 5 6 7 8 Other ________

☐ B.M. ☐ No B.M.

☐ Felt blah ☐ Felt good ♡ Felt great!

Breakfast: Calories ________

Lunch: Calories ________

Dinner: Calories ________

Snacks

Beverages

Notes:

Date: ________ ________ Weight

Daily Details

Today I ate these healthy things:

Today I successfully avoided eating:

I took these supplements:

I Drank this many glasses (8 oz.) of water:

1 2 3 4 5 6 7 8 Other ______

☐ B.M. ☐ No B.M.

☐ Felt blah ☐ Felt good ♡ Felt great!

Breakfast: Calories ________

Lunch: Calories ________

Dinner: Calories ________

Snacks

Beverages

Notes:

Date: ________ ________ Weight

Daily Details

Today I ate these healthy things:

______________________ ______________________

______________________ ______________________

______________________ ______________________

____

Today I successfully avoided eating:

____

____

____

I took these supplements:

____

____

I Drank this many glasses (8 oz.) of water:

1 2 3 4 5 6 7 8 Other ________

☐ B.M. ☐ No B.M.

☐ Felt blah ☐ Felt good ♡ Felt great!

Breakfast: Calories ________

Lunch: Calories ________

Dinner: Calories ________

Snacks

Beverages

Notes:

Date: ________ ________ Weight

Daily Details

Today I ate these healthy things:

Today I successfully avoided eating:

I took these supplements:

I Drank this many glasses (8 oz.) of water:

1 2 3 4 5 6 7 8 Other ________

☐ B.M. ☐ No B.M.

☐ Felt blah ☐ Felt good ♡ Felt great!

Breakfast: Calories ________

Lunch: Calories ________

Dinner: Calories ________

Snacks

Beverages

Notes:

Date: ________ ________ Weight

Daily Details

Today I ate these healthy things:

Today I successfully avoided eating:

I took these supplements:

I Drank this many glasses (8 oz.) of water:

1 2 3 4 5 6 7 8 Other ________

☐ B.M. ☐ No B.M.

☐ Felt blah ☐ Felt good ♡ Felt great!

Breakfast: Calories ________

Lunch: Calories ________

Dinner: Calories ________

Snacks

Beverages

Notes:

Date: ________ ________ Weight

Daily Details

Today I ate these healthy things:

Today I successfully avoided eating:

I took these supplements:

I Drank this many glasses (8 oz.) of water:

1 2 3 4 5 6 7 8 Other ______

☐ B.M. ☐ No B.M.

☐ Felt blah ☐ Felt good ♡ Felt great!

Breakfast: Calories ________

Lunch: Calories ________

Dinner: Calories ________

Snacks

Beverages

Notes:

Date: ________ ________ Weight

Daily Details

Today I ate these healthy things:

Today I successfully avoided eating:

I took these supplements:

I Drank this many glasses (8 oz.) of water:

1 2 3 4 5 6 7 8 Other ______

☐ B.M. ☐ No B.M.

☐ Felt blah ☐ Felt good ♡ Felt great!

Breakfast: Calories ________

Lunch: Calories ________

Dinner: Calories ________

Snacks

Beverages

Notes:

Date: ________ ________ Weight

Daily Details

Today I ate these healthy things:

Today I successfully avoided eating:

I took these supplements:

I Drank this many glasses (8 oz.) of water:

1 2 3 4 5 6 7 8 Other ________

☐ B.M. ☐ No B.M.

☐ Felt blah ☐ Felt good ♡ Felt great!

Breakfast: Calories _______

Lunch: Calories _______

Dinner: Calories _______

Snacks

Beverages

Notes:

Date: ________ ________ Weight

Daily Details

Today I ate these healthy things:

Today I successfully avoided eating:

I took these supplements:

I Drank this many glasses (8 oz.) of water:

1 2 3 4 5 6 7 8 Other ________

☐ B.M. ☐ No B.M.

☐ Felt blah ☐ Felt good ♡ Felt great!

Breakfast: Calories _______

Lunch: Calories _______

Dinner: Calories _______

Snacks

Beverages

Notes:

Date: ________ ________ Weight

Daily Details

Today I ate these healthy things:

Today I successfully avoided eating:

I took these supplements:

I Drank this many glasses (8 oz.) of water:

1 2 3 4 5 6 7 8 Other ________

☐ B.M. ☐ No B.M.

☐ Felt blah ☐ Felt good ♡ Felt great!

Breakfast: Calories ________

Lunch: Calories ________

Dinner: Calories ________

Snacks

Beverages

Notes:

Date: ________ ________ Weight

Daily Details

Today I ate these healthy things:

Today I successfully avoided eating:

I took these supplements:

I Drank this many glasses (8 oz.) of water:

1 2 3 4 5 6 7 8 Other ________

☐ B.M. ☐ No B.M.

☐ Felt blah ☐ Felt good ♡ Felt great!

Breakfast: Calories ______

Lunch: Calories ______

Dinner: Calories ______

Snacks

Beverages

Notes:

Date: ________ ________ Weight

Daily Details

Today I ate these healthy things:

Today I successfully avoided eating:

I took these supplements:

I Drank this many glasses (8 oz.) of water:

1 2 3 4 5 6 7 8 Other ______

☐ B.M. ☐ No B.M.

☐ Felt blah ☐ Felt good ♡ Felt great!

Breakfast: Calories ________

Lunch: Calories ________

Dinner: Calories ________

Snacks

Beverages

Notes:

Date: ________ ________ Weight

Daily Details

Today I ate these healthy things:

Today I successfully avoided eating:

I took these supplements:

I Drank this many glasses (8 oz.) of water:

1 2 3 4 5 6 7 8 Other ________

☐ B.M. ☐ No B.M.

☐ Felt blah ☐ Felt good ♡ Felt great!

Breakfast: Calories ________

Lunch: Calories ________

Dinner: Calories ________

Snacks

Beverages

Notes:

Date: ________ ________ Weight

Daily Details

Today I ate these healthy things:

Today I successfully avoided eating:

I took these supplements:

I Drank this many glasses (8 oz) of water:

1 2 3 4 5 6 7 8 Other ________

☐ B.M. ☐ No B.M.

☐ Felt blah ☐ Felt good ♡ Felt great!

Breakfast: Calories _______

Lunch: Calories _______

Dinner: Calories _______

Snacks

Beverages

Notes:

Date: ________ ________ Weight

Daily Details

Today I ate these healthy things:

Today I successfully avoided eating:

I took these supplements:

I Drank this many glasses (8 oz.) of water:

1 2 3 4 5 6 7 8 Other ________

☐ B.M. ☐ No B.M.

☐ Felt blah ☐ Felt good ♡ Felt great!

Breakfast: Calories ________

Lunch: Calories ________

Dinner: Calories ________

Snacks

Beverages

Notes:

Date: ________ ________ Weight

Daily Details

Today I ate these healthy things:

Today I successfully avoided eating:

I took these supplements:

I Drank this many glasses (8 oz.) of water:

1 2 3 4 5 6 7 8 Other ________

☐ B.M. ☐ No B.M.

☐ Felt blah ☐ Felt good ♡ Felt great!

Breakfast: Calories ________

Lunch: Calories ________

Dinner: Calories ________

Snacks

Beverages

Notes:

Date: ________ ________ Weight

Daily Details

Today I ate these healthy things:

Today I successfully avoided eating:

I took these supplements:

I Drank this many glasses (8 oz.) of water:

1 2 3 4 5 6 7 8 Other ________

☐ B.M. ☐ No B.M.

☐ Felt blah ☐ Felt good ♡ Felt great!

Breakfast: Calories ________

Lunch: Calories ________

Dinner: Calories ________

Snacks

Beverages

Notes:

Date: ________ ________ Weight

Daily Details

Today I ate these healthy things:

Today I successfully avoided eating:

I took these supplements:

I Drank this many glasses (8 oz.) of water:

1 2 3 4 5 6 7 8 Other ________

☐ B.M. ☐ No B.M.

☐ Felt blah ☐ Felt good ♡ Felt great!

Breakfast: Calories _______

Lunch: Calories _______

Dinner: Calories _______

Snacks

Beverages

Notes:

Date: ________ ________ Weight

Daily Details

Today I ate these healthy things:

Today I successfully avoided eating:

I took these supplements:

I Drank this many glasses (8 oz.) of water:

1 2 3 4 5 6 7 8 Other ________

☐ B.M. ☐ No B.M.

☐ Felt blah ☐ Felt good ♡ Felt great!

Breakfast: Calories ________

Lunch: Calories ________

Dinner: Calories ________

Snacks

Beverages

Notes:

Date: ________ ________ Weight

Daily Details

Today I ate these healthy things:

Today I successfully avoided eating:

I took these supplements:

I Drank this many glasses (8 oz.) of water:

1 2 3 4 5 6 7 8 Other ________

☐ B.M. ☐ No B.M.

☐ Felt blah ☐ Felt good ♡ Felt great!

Breakfast: Calories ________

Lunch: Calories ________

Dinner: Calories ________

Snacks

Beverages

Notes:

Date: ________ ________ Weight

Daily Details

Today I ate these healthy things:

Today I successfully avoided eating:

I took these supplements:

I Drank this many glasses (8 oz.) of water:

1 2 3 4 5 6 7 8 Other ________

☐ B.M. ☐ No B.M.

☐ Felt blah ☐ Felt good ♡ Felt great!

Breakfast: Calories ________

Lunch: Calories ________

Dinner: Calories ________

Snacks

Beverages

Notes:

Date: ________ ________ Weight

Daily Details

Today I ate these healthy things:

Today I successfully avoided eating:

I took these supplements:

I Drank this many glasses (8 oz.) of water:

1 2 3 4 5 6 7 8 Other ________

☐ B.M. ☐ No B.M.

☐ Felt blah ☐ Felt good ♡ Felt great!

Breakfast: Calories ________

Lunch: Calories ________

Dinner: Calories ________

Snacks

Beverages

Notes:

Date: ________ ________ Weight

Daily Details

Today I ate these healthy things:

Today I successfully avoided eating:

I took these supplements:

I Drank this many glasses (8 oz) of water:

1 2 3 4 5 6 7 8 Other ________

☐ B.M. ☐ No B.M.

☐ Felt blah ☐ Felt good ♡ Felt great!

Breakfast: Calories ________

Lunch: Calories ________

Dinner: Calories ________

Snacks

Beverages

Notes:

Date: ________ ________ Weight

Daily Details

Today I ate these healthy things:

Today I successfully avoided eating:

I took these supplements:

I Drank this many glasses (8 oz.) of water:

1 2 3 4 5 6 7 8 Other ________

☐ B.M. ☐ No B.M.

☐ Felt blah ☐ Felt good ♡ Felt great!

Breakfast: Calories ________

Lunch: Calories ________

Dinner: Calories ________

Snacks

Beverages

Notes:

Date: ________ ________ Weight

Daily Details

Today I ate these healthy things:

Today I successfully avoided eating:

I took these supplements:

I Drank this many glasses (8 oz.) of water:

1 2 3 4 5 6 7 8 Other ________

☐ B.M. ☐ No B.M.

☐ Felt blah ☐ Felt good ♡ Felt great!

Breakfast: Calories ________

Lunch: Calories ________

Dinner: Calories ________

Snacks

Beverages

Notes:

Date: ________ ________ Weight

Daily Details

Today I ate these healthy things:

Today I successfully avoided eating:

I took these supplements:

I Drank this many glasses (8 oz.) of water:

1 2 3 4 5 6 7 8 Other ________

☐ B.M. ☐ No B.M.

☐ Felt blah ☐ Felt good ♡ Felt great!

Breakfast: Calories ______

Lunch: Calories ______

Dinner: Calories ______

Snacks

Beverages

Notes:

Date: ________ ________ Weight

Daily Details

Today I ate these healthy things:

Today I successfully avoided eating:

I took these supplements:

I Drank this many glasses (8 oz.) of water:

1 2 3 4 5 6 7 8 Other ________

☐ B.M. ☐ No B.M.

☐ Felt blah ☐ Felt good ♡ Felt great!

Breakfast: Calories ________

Lunch: Calories ________

Dinner: Calories ________

Snacks

Beverages

Notes:

Date: ________ ________ Weight

Daily Details

Today I ate these healthy things:

Today I successfully avoided eating:

I took these supplements:

I Drank this many glasses (8 oz.) of water:

1 2 3 4 5 6 7 8 Other ________

☐ B.M. ☐ No B.M.

☐ Felt blah ☐ Felt good ♡ Felt great!

Breakfast: Calories ________

Lunch: Calories ________

Dinner: Calories ________

Snacks

Beverages

Notes:

Date: ________ ________ Weight

Daily Details

Today I ate these healthy things:

Today I successfully avoided eating:

I took these supplements:

I Drank this many glasses (8 oz.) of water:

1 2 3 4 5 6 7 8 Other ________

☐ B.M. ☐ No B.M.

☐ Felt blah ☐ Felt good ♡ Felt great!

Breakfast: Calories ________

Lunch: Calories ________

Dinner: Calories ________

Snacks

Beverages

Notes:

Date: ________ ________ Weight

Daily Details

Today I ate these healthy things:

Today I successfully avoided eating:

I took these supplements:

I Drank this many glasses (8 oz.) of water:

1 2 3 4 5 6 7 8 Other ________

☐ B.M. ☐ No B.M.

☐ Felt blah ☐ Felt good ♡ Felt great!

Breakfast: Calories ________

Lunch: Calories ________

Dinner: Calories ________

Snacks

Beverages

Notes:

Date: ________ ________ Weight

Daily Details

Today I ate these healthy things:

Today I successfully avoided eating:

I took these supplements:

I Drank this many glasses (8 oz.) of water:

1 2 3 4 5 6 7 8 Other ______

☐ B.M. ☐ No B.M.

☐ Felt blah ☐ Felt good ♡ Felt great!

Breakfast: Calories ______

Lunch: Calories ______

Dinner: Calories ______

Snacks

Beverages

Notes:

Date: ________ ________ Weight

Daily Details

Today I ate these healthy things:

Today I successfully avoided eating:

I took these supplements:

I Drank this many glasses (8 oz.) of water:

1 2 3 4 5 6 7 8 Other ______

☐ B.M. ☐ No B.M.

☐ Felt blah ☐ Felt good ♡ Felt great!

Breakfast: Calories ________

Lunch: Calories ________

Dinner: Calories ________

Snacks

Beverages

Notes:

Date: ________ ________ Weight

Daily Details

Today I ate these healthy things:

Today I successfully avoided eating:

I took these supplements:

I Drank this many glasses (8 oz.) of water:

1 2 3 4 5 6 7 8 Other ______

☐ B.M. ☐ No B.M.

☐ Felt blah ☐ Felt good ♡ Felt great!

Breakfast: Calories ________

Lunch: Calories ________

Dinner: Calories ________

Snacks

Beverages

Notes:

Date: ________ ________ Weight

Daily Details

Today I ate these healthy things:

Today I successfully avoided eating:

I took these supplements:

I Drank this many glasses (8 oz.) of water:

1 2 3 4 5 6 7 8 Other ________

☐ B.M. ☐ No B.M.

☐ Felt blah ☐ Felt good ♡ Felt great!

Breakfast: Calories ______

Lunch: Calories ______

Dinner: Calories ______

Snacks

Beverages

Notes:

Date: ________ ________ Weight

Daily Details

Today I ate these healthy things:

Today I successfully avoided eating:

I took these supplements:

I Drank this many glasses (8 oz.) of water:

1 2 3 4 5 6 7 8 Other ________

☐ B.M. ☐ No B.M.

☐ Felt blah ☐ Felt good ♡ Felt great!

Breakfast: Calories _______

Lunch: Calories _______

Dinner: Calories _______

Snacks

Beverages

Notes:

Date: __________ __________ Weight

Daily Details

Today I ate these healthy things:

Today I successfully avoided eating:

I took these supplements:

I Drank this many glasses (8 oz.) of water:

1 2 3 4 5 6 7 8 Other __________

☐ B.M. ☐ No B.M.

☐ Felt blah ☐ Felt good ♡ Felt great!

Breakfast: Calories ________

Lunch: Calories ________

Dinner: Calories ________

Snacks

Beverages

Notes:

Date: ________ ________ Weight

Daily Details

Today I ate these healthy things:

Today I successfully avoided eating:

I took these supplements:

I Drank this many glasses (8 oz.) of water:

1 2 3 4 5 6 7 8 Other ________

☐ B.M. ☐ No B.M.

☐ Felt blah ☐ Felt good ♡ Felt great!

Breakfast: Calories ________

Lunch: Calories ________

Dinner: Calories ________

Snacks

Beverages

Notes:

Date: ________ ________ Weight

Daily Details

Today I ate these healthy things:

Today I successfully avoided eating:

I took these supplements:

I Drank this many glasses (8 oz) of water:

1 2 3 4 5 6 7 8 Other ________

☐ B.M. ☐ No B.M.

☐ Felt blah ☐ Felt good ♡ Felt great!

Breakfast: Calories ________

Lunch: Calories ________

Dinner: Calories ________

Snacks

Beverages

Notes:

Date: ________ ________ Weight

Daily Details

Today I ate these healthy things:

Today I successfully avoided eating:

I took these supplements:

I Drank this many glasses (8 oz.) of water:

1 2 3 4 5 6 7 8 Other ________

☐ B.M. ☐ No B.M.

☐ Felt blah ☐ Felt good ♡ Felt great!

Breakfast: Calories ________

Lunch: Calories ________

Dinner: Calories ________

Snacks

Beverages

Notes:

Date: ________ ________ Weight

Daily Details

Today I ate these healthy things:

Today I successfully avoided eating:

I took these supplements:

I Drank this many glasses (8 oz.) of water:

1 2 3 4 5 6 7 8 Other ______

☐ B.M. ☐ No B.M.

☐ Felt blah ☐ Felt good ♡ Felt great!

Breakfast: Calories ________

Lunch: Calories ________

Dinner: Calories ________

Snacks

Beverages

Notes:

Date: ________ ________ Weight

Daily Details

Today I ate these healthy things:

Today I successfully avoided eating:

I took these supplements:

I Drank this many glasses (8 oz.) of water:

1 2 3 4 5 6 7 8 Other ________

☐ B.M. ☐ No B.M.

☐ Felt blah ☐ Felt good ♡ Felt great!

Breakfast: Calories ________

Lunch: Calories ________

Dinner: Calories ________

Snacks

Beverages

Notes:

Date: ________ ________ Weight

Daily Details

Today I ate these healthy things:

Today I successfully avoided eating:

I took these supplements:

I Drank this many glasses (8 oz.) of water:

1 2 3 4 5 6 7 8 Other ________

☐ B.M. ☐ No B.M.

☐ Felt blah ☐ Felt good ♡ Felt great!

Breakfast: Calories ________

Lunch: Calories ________

Dinner: Calories ________

Snacks

Beverages

Notes:

Date: ________ ________ Weight

Daily Details

Today I ate these healthy things:

Today I successfully avoided eating:

I took these supplements:

I Drank this many glasses (8 oz.) of water:

1 2 3 4 5 6 7 8 Other ________

☐ B.M. ☐ No B.M.

☐ Felt blah ☐ Felt good ♡ Felt great!

Breakfast: Calories ________

Lunch: Calories ________

Dinner: Calories ________

Snacks

Beverages

Notes:

Date: ________ ________ Weight

Daily Details

Today I ate these healthy things:

Today I successfully avoided eating:

I took these supplements:

I Drank this many glasses (8 oz.) of water:

1 2 3 4 5 6 7 8 Other ________

☐ B.M. ☐ No B.M.

☐ Felt blah ☐ Felt good ♡ Felt great!

Breakfast: Calories _______

Lunch: Calories _______

Dinner: Calories _______

Snacks

Beverages

Notes:

Date: ________ ________ Weight

Daily Details

Today I ate these healthy things:

Today I successfully avoided eating:

I took these supplements:

I Drank this many glasses (8 oz.) of water:

1 2 3 4 5 6 7 8 Other ________

☐ B.M. ☐ No B.M.

☐ Felt blah ☐ Felt good ♡ Felt great!

Breakfast: Calories ________

Lunch: Calories ________

Dinner: Calories ________

Snacks

Beverages

Notes:

Date: ________ ________ Weight

Daily Details

Today I ate these healthy things:

Today I successfully avoided eating:

I took these supplements:

I Drank this many glasses (8 oz) of water:

1 2 3 4 5 6 7 8 Other ________

☐ B.M. ☐ No B.M.

☐ Felt blah ☐ Felt good ♡ Felt great!

Breakfast: Calories ________

Lunch: Calories ________

Dinner: Calories ________

Snacks

Beverages

Notes:

Date: ________ ________ Weight

Daily Details

Today I ate these healthy things:

Today I successfully avoided eating:

I took these supplements:

I Drank this many glasses (8 oz.) of water:

1 2 3 4 5 6 7 8 Other ________

☐ B.M. ☐ No B.M.

☐ Felt blah ☐ Felt good ♡ Felt great!

Breakfast: Calories ______

Lunch: Calories ______

Dinner: Calories ______

Snacks

Beverages

Notes:

Date: ________ ________ Weight

Daily Details

Today I ate these healthy things:

Today I successfully avoided eating:

I took these supplements:

I Drank this many glasses (8 oz.) of water:

1 2 3 4 5 6 7 8 Other ________

☐ B.M. ☐ No B.M.

☐ Felt blah ☐ Felt good ♡ Felt great!

Breakfast: Calories ________

Lunch: Calories ________

Dinner: Calories ________

Snacks

Beverages

Notes:

Date: ________ ________ Weight

Daily Details

Today I ate these healthy things:

Today I successfully avoided eating:

I took these supplements:

I Drank this many glasses (8 oz.) of water:

1 2 3 4 5 6 7 8 Other ________

☐ B.M. ☐ No B.M.

☐ Felt blah ☐ Felt good ♡ Felt great!

Breakfast: Calories _______

Lunch: Calories _______

Dinner: Calories _______

Snacks

Beverages

Notes:

Date: ________ ________ Weight

Daily Details

Today I ate these healthy things:

Today I successfully avoided eating:

I took these supplements:

I Drank this many glasses (8 oz.) of water:

1 2 3 4 5 6 7 8 Other ________

☐ B.M. ☐ No B.M.

☐ Felt blah ☐ Felt good ♡ Felt great!

Breakfast: Calories ________

Lunch: Calories ________

Dinner: Calories ________

Snacks

Beverages

Notes:

Made in the USA
Monee, IL
04 November 2026

67375673R00108